# A FRESH START

## Cancer-Fighting Recipes for the Newly Diagnosed

## Aaliyah Briggs

# TABLE OF CONTENTS

# INTRODUCTION

Once upon a time, there was a prosperous businessman named John. He led a fast-paced life and was constantly on the move. However, one day he received some devastating news. He was diagnosed with cancer by his doctor. John was devastated and thought his life was over.

But John was adamant about not giving up. He had always heard that eating the right foods could help you fight off illnesses, so he decided to make a change. He began eating a well-balanced diet rich in fruits and vegetables, whole grains, and lean proteins. He also made an effort to drink plenty of water and limit his intake of processed foods and sugar.

John began to feel better as he adhered to his new diet. His energy levels increased, and he was able to sleep better at night. After a few weeks, his doctor informed him that his cancer had begun to shrink and that he was on the mend.

John was overjoyed and continued with his new healthy lifestyle. He even began to share his story with others, encouraging them to make the same changes that had helped him. He was an inspiration to many, and his positive attitude and determination to fight his cancer inspired others to live healthier lives.

In the end, John was able to beat his cancer and live a long, healthy life. He was grateful for the power of good nutrition and the impact it had on his life. He was living proof that a healthy diet can truly make a difference in the fight against cancer.

# CHAPTER 1

## What Is Cancer?

Cancer is a class of diseases distinguished by abnormal cell growth. It can affect any part of the body and is characterized by uncontrolled cell growth that can spread to other parts of the body. Tumors, pain, and other symptoms can be caused by the growth and spread of cancer cells. Cancer treatment may include surgery, chemotherapy, radiation, and immunotherapy.

Cancer is a group of hundreds of different diseases. Breast cancer, lung cancer, prostate cancer, colon cancer, and lymphoma are common types.

## Different Types of Cancer

**1. Carcinoma:** A carcinoma is a type of cancer that begins in the tissues that line organs such as the lungs, breasts, pancreas, and colon. Carcinomas are the most common type of cancer and involve the uncontrolled growth of cells in the lining of these organs.

**2. Sarcoma:** Sarcoma is a type of cancer that begins in connective tissues such as muscles, fat, blood vessels, and cartilage. Sarcomas are less common than carcinomas and often more aggressive, making them difficult to treat.

**3. Lymphoma:** Lymphoma is a type of cancer that begins in lymphocytes, which are white blood cells. Lymphomas can be Hodgkin's or non-Hodgkin's. They can affect any part of the body and grow slowly or quickly.

**4. Leukemia:** Leukemia is a type of cancer that begins in the blood and bone marrow. The uncontrolled growth of abnormal white blood cells causes it. Acute leukemias develop and progress quickly, whereas chronic leukemias develop slowly over time.

**5. Melanoma:** Melanoma is a type of skin cancer that begins in the cells that give skin its color. It is one of the most dangerous and aggressive types of skin cancer and is frequently caused by UV light exposure. Early detection is critical for successful treatment.

**6. Brain Tumor:** A brain tumor is a type of cancer that begins in the brain or surrounding tissues. Brain tumors can be benign (not cancerous) or malignant (cancerous) (cancerous). Brain tumors can cause a variety of symptoms depending on where the tumor is located.

**7. Thyroid:** Thyroid cancer is a type of cancer that begins in the thyroid gland. It is usually caused by a genetic mutation and can be either slow-growing or aggressive. It is more common in women and can be treated with surgery, radiation, and hormone therapy.

Early detection and treatment are critical to improving outcomes regardless of the type of cancer. It is critical to understand the various types of cancer and to consult your doctor if you are experiencing any symptoms.

# Cancer Causes and Risk Factors

Cancer is a multifaceted disease caused by a variety of factors. It happens when normal cells in the body grow and divide uncontrollably, resulting in a mass of cells known as a tumor. Cancer can occur in virtually any part of the body, including the skin, bones, organs, and tissues.

Cancer's exact causes are unknown, but several factors have been identified as contributing to its development. Cancer's primary causes and risk factors include:

1. **Genetics:** Certain types of cancer are more likely to develop as a result of genetic mutations. Mutations in the BRCA1 and BRCA2 genes, for example, increase the risk of breast and ovarian cancer.

2. **Environmental factors**: Certain chemicals, radiation, and pollutants have been linked to an increased risk of cancer. Tobacco smoke, for

example, contains more than 70 carcinogenic chemicals and is a leading cause of lung cancer.

3. **Infections:** Cancer can be caused by certain viruses and bacteria. Human papillomavirus (HPV), for example, can cause cervical cancer, and hepatitis B and C viruses can cause liver cancer.

4. **Lifestyle factors:** Certain lifestyle choices, such as a poor diet, lack of physical activity, and excessive alcohol consumption, can increase the risk of cancer.

5. **Age:** Cancer risk increases with age. The majority of cancers are discovered in people over the age of 50.

6. **Gender:** Certain cancers, such as breast and prostate cancer, are more common in women than in men.

7. **Family history:** If a close relative has been diagnosed with cancer, you may be at a higher risk of developing the disease.

8. **Medical history:** People who have had cancer in the past are more likely to develop it again.

It is critical to understand that having one or more of these risk factors does not guarantee that a person will develop cancer. Some people who have a lot of risk factors never get the disease, while others who have few or no risk factors do.

It is also important to understand that some cancers can be avoided or detected early through lifestyle changes, regular cancer screenings, and appropriate medical care.

## Cancer and Diet

If you have recently been diagnosed with cancer, you should know how diet can help you manage your condition. Eating a healthy, well-balanced diet can help you maintain your health, manage treatment side effects, and lower your risk of developing other health issues.

Begin by consulting with your doctor or a dietitian to create a meal plan that works for you. Fresh fruits and vegetables, whole grains, and lean proteins like fish, chicken, and beans should all be part of your diet. Reduce your intake of processed foods and foods high in sugar, salt, and saturated fats. You should also consume enough fiber and fluids.

Your diet should prioritize the provision of essential nutrients to your body, such as vitamins, minerals, and antioxidants. Consuming antioxidant-rich foods, such as dark green and orange vegetables, may help reduce your risk of cancer recurrence. Eating calcium-rich foods, such as dairy products and dark leafy greens, may also be beneficial.

It's important to remember that everyone's nutritional needs are different, so talk to your doctor or a dietitian before making any major dietary changes. Additionally, discuss any supplements you are thinking about taking with your doctor. Supplements can be beneficial, but they can also be harmful if not taken under the supervision of a doctor.

Finally, living a healthy lifestyle can assist you in managing your cancer. Regular exercise, adequate sleep, and stress reduction can all help you maintain your health and lower your chances of recurrence of cancer.

Understanding the role of diet in cancer management allows you to take steps to ensure that you are getting the essential nutrients that your body requires to stay healthy.

## Importance of a Healthy Diet During Cancer Treatment

A healthy, balanced diet is an essential part of cancer treatment. Eating the right foods can help patients maintain their strength, deal with side effects, and fight infections. A healthy diet can also help reduce the risk of developing other health problems while undergoing cancer treatment.

A healthy diet can help the body heal and deal with the side effects of cancer treatments like chemotherapy and radiation therapy. Eating a variety of nutrient-dense foods can help boost energy, reduce fatigue, and maintain a healthy weight. A healthy diet can also help to reduce nausea, vomiting, and diarrhea.

A healthy diet can also help the body fight infections and maintain a strong immune system. Protein, vitamins, minerals, and antioxidant-rich foods can help the body fight infection and heal faster. Drinking plenty of fluids is also important for keeping the body hydrated and flushing out toxins.

A healthy diet can help reduce the risk of developing other health problems while undergoing cancer treatment. A diet high in fiber and low in saturated fat can help reduce the risk of developing diabetes, heart disease, and other chronic diseases. A diet high in fruits and vegetables can also help reduce the risk of developing certain cancers.

Eating a healthy diet while undergoing cancer treatment can be difficult, especially if patients are experiencing nausea, vomiting, or diarrhea. However, it is still necessary to make an effort to eat nutritious, balanced meals in order to aid the body's recovery and defense against infections. Eating the right foods can help patients maintain their strength and lower their chances of developing other health issues.

A healthy diet is an important part of the recovery process during cancer treatment. Eating a variety of nutritious foods can aid in healing, coping with side effects, and lowering the risk of developing other health issues. Patients should consult their doctor or a dietitian for more information on eating a healthy diet while undergoing cancer treatment.

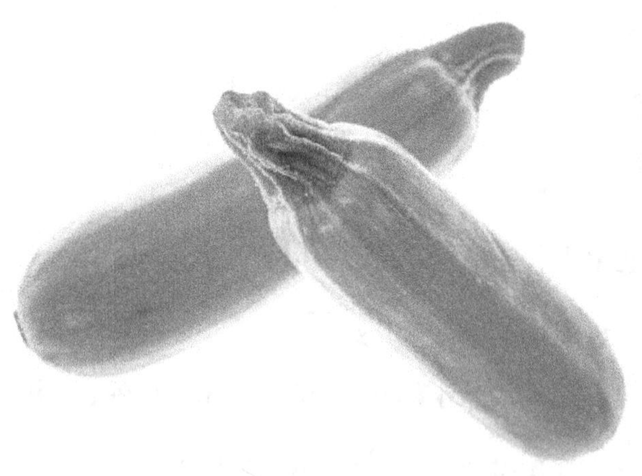

# CHAPTER 2

## The Science Behind Food and Cancer

Humans have long relied on food for sustenance, pleasure, and comfort. However, it has recently become a source of interest as researchers investigate the possible links between diet and cancer.

The notion that what we eat can have an impact on our health is not new. Nutritionists and doctors have been warning us for years to avoid certain foods, such as those high in fat and sugar, and to stick to a nutritious diet. But how does food influence cancer risk?

Food, at its most basic, provides us with the energy and nutrients we require to maintain our health. However, some foods may contain cancer-causing agents, such as pesticides, which can accumulate in the body over time and potentially initiate tumor development.

Furthermore, certain vitamins and minerals may act as antioxidants, which can help to protect cells from free radical damage. For example, studies suggest that diets high in carotenoid-rich foods like carrots, spinach, and sweet potatoes may lower the risk of certain cancers.

Furthermore, certain foods may contain substances that stimulate the body's natural defense mechanisms and kill cancer cells. Cruciferous vegetables, such as broccoli and Brussels sprouts, contain glucosinolates, which can activate enzymes that aid the body's fight against cancer.

Finally, some foods may contain natural compounds that can aid in the reduction of inflammation, which is thought to play a role in the development of some cancers. Omega-3 fatty acids, found in foods like salmon and walnuts, for example, have been shown to reduce inflammation in the body.

The science of food and cancer is still in its early stages. However, it is clear that what we eat can affect our overall health and our risk of developing certain diseases, such as cancer. As a result, it's critical to eat nutrient-dense foods and avoid processed and sugary foods as much as possible.

## Understanding the Nutritional Role in Cancer

Cancer prevention and treatment rely heavily on nutrition. A healthy diet, a healthy weight, and regular physical activity can all help reduce the risk of developing certain types of cancer. A balanced diet can also help cancer patients manage their symptoms and improve their quality of life.

By providing the body with essential vitamins and minerals, as well as other nutrients, good nutrition can help reduce the risk of cancer. Eating a variety of healthy foods high in antioxidants can help protect the body from free radical damage. Eating high-fiber foods can also help reduce the risk of certain types of cancer, including colorectal cancer.

Maintaining a healthy weight is also important for lowering cancer risk. Excess body fat has been linked to an increased risk of certain cancers, including breast and colorectal cancer. Eating a well-balanced diet and engaging in regular physical activity can help you maintain a healthy weight and lower your risk of cancer.

Cancer patients can benefit from good nutrition as well. A healthy diet can help the body get the energy it needs to fight the disease. Protein-rich foods can help cancer patients maintain muscle mass and strength, which is important for those undergoing chemotherapy. Additionally, eating foods high in fiber can help reduce chemotherapy side effects such as nausea and diarrhea.

Good nutrition can help cancer patients improve their quality of life. A healthy diet can make cancer patients feel better and give them more energy.

Nutrition is critical in the prevention and treatment of cancer. A healthy diet, a healthy weight, and regular physical activity can all help reduce the risk of cancer.

Furthermore, good nutrition can assist cancer patients in managing their symptoms and improving their quality of life.

## The Link Between Certain Foods and Cancer

A growing body of evidence suggests that diet plays a role in cancer development. A diet high in fruits and vegetables, whole grains, and lean meats have been shown in studies to reduce the risk of certain types of cancer. Diets high in processed meats, sugar, and saturated fats, on the other hand, may increase the risk of certain types of cancer.

For decades, scientists have investigated the link between certain foods and cancer. They discovered that certain food components may increase the risk of cancer. Processed meats, for example, contain nitrates and nitrites, which can combine to form cancer-causing compounds in the body. Red and processed meat consumption have been linked to an increased risk of colorectal cancer.

Furthermore, high-sugar and saturated-fat diets may increase the risk of certain types of cancer. Sugar consumption has been linked to an increased risk of breast and endometrial cancer, while a high-fat diet has been linked to an increased risk of prostate and colon cancer.

The good news is that certain foods may help lower the risk of cancer. Antioxidants found in fruits and vegetables help protect cells from damage that can lead to cancer. Whole grains are also beneficial because they contain fiber, which can help reduce inflammation and the risk of cancer in the body. Eating lean proteins like fish, chicken, and beans can also help lower your risk of cancer.

The link between certain foods and cancer is becoming clearer. A diet high in fruits and vegetables, whole grains, and lean proteins may lower the risk of certain types of cancer, whereas processed meats, sugar, and saturated fats may increase the risk. It is critical to focus on eating a variety of healthy foods for optimal health and cancer prevention.

## Certain Foods Have Anticancer Properties

A diet rich in these foods may reduce the risk of cancer and improve overall health, according to growing evidence. Here are a couple of examples:

1. **Berries:** Berries rich in antioxidants, such as strawberries, blueberries, and raspberries, can help protect cells from damage that can lead to cancer. Berries also contain anti-inflammatory compounds, which may aid in the reduction of inflammation in the body, which is yet another risk factor for cancer.

2. **Cruciferous vegetables include:** Cruciferous vegetables, such as broccoli, cabbage, and kale, are high in glucosinolates, which are broken down in the body to form active compounds that can aid in cancer prevention. These vegetables also contain a

lot of fiber, which has been linked to a lower risk of colorectal cancer.

3. **Garlic:** Garlic is a kitchen staple known for its potent antibacterial and antiviral properties. It has also been shown to have anticancer properties, most likely due to the presence of compounds such as allicin, which can aid in the prevention of cancer cell growth.

4. **Tomatoes:** Tomatoes are high in lycopene, a powerful antioxidant linked to a lower risk of prostate cancer. Lycopene may also help prevent other types of cancer, such as lung, breast, and stomach cancer, according to research.

5. **Green tea:** Green tea contains a high concentration of polyphenols, which have been shown to have anticancer properties. Polyphenol EGCG (epigallocatechin gallate) in particular has been shown to have a powerful effect on cancer cells, preventing them from growing and spreading.

These are just a few of the many foods with anticancer properties that have been discovered. Eating a healthy diet rich in these foods may help to reduce the risk of cancer and may even help to treat it.

While these foods have been shown to have potential anticancer properties, they should not be used as the sole method of cancer prevention. A healthy diet and lifestyle, including regular exercise and quitting smoking, are the most effective ways to lower your cancer risk and improve your overall health.

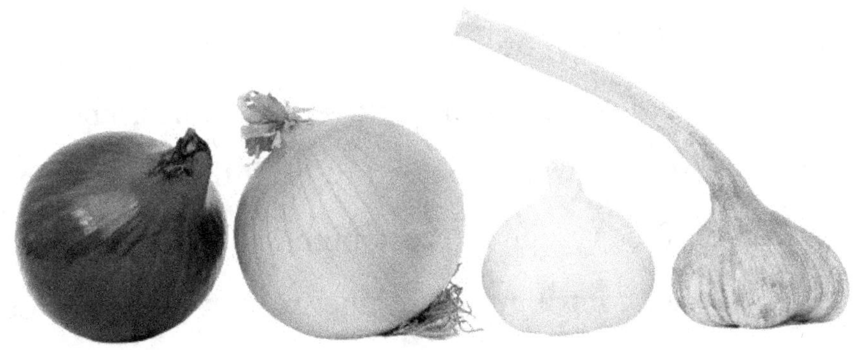

# CHAPTER 3

## The Importance of Meal Planning

Meal planning can be critical to a newly diagnosed cancer patient's recovery and overall well-being. Proper nutrition is necessary for maintaining strength, fighting infections, and assisting the body in healing. A well-planned diet can also help manage treatment symptoms and side effects such as nausea and fatigue.

It is critical for cancer patients to focus on a diet that provides adequate energy and essential nutrients. This could include eating more lean meats, poultry, fish, beans, and dairy products, as well as foods high in vitamins and minerals like fruits, vegetables, and whole grains. Patients may also need to limit their consumption of certain foods, such as those high in sugar, salt, and fat, as these can contribute to fatigue, weight gain, and other health issues.

Meal planning can assist cancer patients in better managing their diet by ensuring they always have healthy, balanced meals available. This can include creating menus, making grocery lists, and preparing meals ahead of time. Planning ahead of time can also help patients stick to their dietary goals, even on hectic days when they may not have time to cook.

A meal plan can also assist cancer patients in managing their symptoms and the side effects of treatment. Some cancer patients, for example, may experience nausea or vomiting, making it difficult to eat. A meal plan can assist these patients in prioritizing foods that they can tolerate better, such as clear liquids or bland, high-protein snacks.

To summarize, meal planning is an important tool for cancer patients to use to support their physical and emotional health as they recover. Patients can develop a customized meal plan that meets their specific needs and helps them feel their best with the assistance of a healthcare professional or a registered dietitian.

# Tips for Easier Meal Preparation

Meal preparation can be difficult for anyone, but it can be especially difficult for a cancer patient who has recently been diagnosed. The physical and emotional toll of the diagnosis, combined with the side effects of treatment, can make it difficult to even consider cooking. However, because proper nutrition is important for managing cancer symptoms and supporting overall health, it's critical to find ways to make meal preparation easier.

Here are some guides to get you started:

1. **Make a plan:** Making a weekly meal plan can help take some of the stress out of meal preparation. Make a grocery list based on what you intend to cook for each meal. This way, you'll have everything you need and won't have to think about what to make every day.

2. **Maintain simplicity:** Complex meals can be overwhelming, especially if you lack energy.

Soups, stews, and salads are examples of simple, nourishing meals that can be easily prepared.

3. **Preparation in bulk:** Meal preparation ahead of time can save time and energy later. On weekends, make a large batch of food and freeze individual portions for later. All you have to do when you're ready to eat is reheat.

4. **Purchase kitchen appliances:** Meal preparation can be simplified by using a slow cooker, pressure cooker, or instant pot. These appliances can cook food quickly and efficiently, giving you more time and energy to devote to other activities.

5. **Make use of pre-cut and pre-washed produce:** Purchasing pre-cut and pre-washed produce can help you save time and stress. This allows you to spend less time chopping and washing and more time cooking and eating a nutritious meal.

6. **Ask for help:** Don't be afraid to seek assistance from friends and family. They may be able to assist you with meal preparation, grocery shopping, or even running errands.

**7. Consult a dietitian:** A registered dietitian can assist you in developing a meal plan that meets your specific needs while also assisting you in managing cancer symptoms. They can also offer suggestions on how to make meal preparation simpler and more manageable.

Making meal preparation easier for newly diagnosed cancer patients can benefit their overall health and quality of life. They can focus on their health and healing while still enjoying nourishing and delicious meals if they follow these tips.

## Essential Kitchen Tools and Utensils

If you have recently been diagnosed with cancer, it is critical to stock your kitchen with the necessary tools and utensils to make meal preparation easier and healthier. Here are a few kitchen tools and utensils that every cancer patient should have:

**1. High-Quality Knives:** All cancer patients should invest in a high-quality knife set. When it comes to


Cancer-Fighting Recipes for the Newly Diagnosed

chopping and slicing ingredients for meals, high-quality knives will make your life much easier.

**2. Vegetable Peeler:** All cancer patients should have a vegetable peeler. Peeling vegetables can help reduce the risk of ingesting harmful toxins found on or inside the skin of certain vegetables.

**3. Cutting Board:** Having a cutting board in your kitchen is essential for reducing the risk of cross-contamination. Invest in a high-quality cutting board that will not dull your knives and is easy to clean.

**4. Blender:** Use a blender to make smoothies and other healthy drinks. Blenders can also be used to puree soups and sauces.

**5. Measuring Cups and Spoons:** When it comes to cooking and baking, precise measurements are essential. Purchasing a set of measuring cups and spoons will assist you in obtaining accurate measurements for all of your recipes.

**6. Food Processor:** A food processor is an excellent tool for cancer patients because it allows for quick and easy chopping and pureeing of ingredients. This can greatly simplify and expedite meal preparation.

**7. Slow Cooker:** If you don't have the energy to stand and cook, a slow cooker can be a great way to prepare meals quickly. Slow cookers are ideal for making nutritious soups, stews, and other dishes.

**8. Nonstick Cookware:** Having nonstick cookware can help cancer patients reduce the amount of fat and oil that is required to cook meals. Nonstick cookware also makes cleanup easier.

These are just a few of the necessary kitchen tools and utensils for a newly diagnosed cancer patient's kitchen. You can ensure that you have everything you need to prepare nutritious and delicious meals by investing in the right kitchen tools and utensils.

# CHAPTER 4

## Seven (7) days Meal plan with instructions

## Day 1

**Breakfast:** Oatmeal with berries and nuts for breakfast.

**Instructions:** Mix together ½ cup of cooked oatmeal, a handful of fresh berries, a tablespoon of chopped nuts, and a tablespoon of honey.

**Lunch:** Soup with lentils and vegetables

**Instructions:** Sauté one diced onion, one diced bell pepper, and two cloves of minced garlic in a tablespoon of extra-virgin olive oil in a large pot over medium heat. Combine two cups of cooked lentils, four cups of vegetable broth, and one teaspoon of dried oregano in a mixing bowl. Cook for 15 minutes.

**Dinner:** Baked fish with steamed vegetables

**Instructions:** Preheat the oven to 375 degrees Fahrenheit. On a baking sheet, place a 6-ounce filet of fish. Add a teaspoon of olive oil, a squeeze of lemon juice, and a pinch of salt and pepper to taste. 15 minutes in the oven. Steam 1 cup broccoli and 1 cup cauliflower for 8 minutes while the fish bakes.

**Snacks:** Hummus and vegetables.

**Instructions:** In a food processor, combine one can of chickpeas, two cloves of garlic, two tablespoons of tahini, and one teaspoon of lemon juice. Blend until smooth. Serve alongside sliced vegetables.

**Dessert:** Chocolate-dipped strawberries.

**Instructions:** Melt 1 cup of dark chocolate chips in a double boiler over low heat. Place fresh strawberries on parchment paper after dipping them in melted chocolate. Cool until the chocolate has hardened.

**Smoothie:** blueberries, bananas, and almond milk.

**Instructions:** In a blender, combine 1 cup of almond milk, 1 banana, 1 cup of frozen blueberries, a handful of spinach, and 1 tablespoon of honey. Blend until completely smooth.

## Day 2

**Breakfast:** Egg and vegetable scramble.

**Instructions:** In a mixing bowl, whisk together two eggs. In a skillet over medium heat, heat 1 tablespoon of extra-virgin olive oil. Cook for 5 minutes after adding one cup of diced vegetables (such as bell peppers and mushrooms). Scramble the eggs until they are cooked through.

**Lunch:** Quinoa and black bean bowl.

**Instructions:** In a mixing bowl, combine 1 cup of cooked quinoa, 1 cup of cooked black beans, ½ cup of diced tomatoes, 1 tablespoon of chopped cilantro, and 1 tablespoon of lime juice.

**Dinner:** Grilled chicken and roasted vegetables.

**Instructions:** Preheat the oven to 425 degrees Fahrenheit. Toss one cup of chopped vegetables (such as zucchini and bell peppers) with one tablespoon of olive oil and a pinch of salt and pepper in a mixing bowl. Cook for 20 minutes at 350°F. Meanwhile, salt and pepper one 6-ounce chicken breast. Cook the chicken for 8 minutes per side in a skillet with a tablespoon of olive oil over medium heat.

**Snacks:** Greek yogurt and granola.

**Instructions:** Top a cup of nonfat Greek yogurt with a tablespoon of granola and a handful of berries.

**Dessert:** Baked apples.

**Instructions:** Preheat the oven to 375 degrees Fahrenheit. Place two apples in a baking dish and core them. Fill a tablespoon of brown sugar, one teaspoon of butter, and a sprinkle of cinnamon into the center of each apple. Cook for 20 minutes.

**Smoothie:** Avocado, spinach, and almond milk.

**Instructions:** In a blender, combine one cup of almond milk, ½ avocado, One cup of spinach, one banana, and one tablespoon of honey. Blend until completely smooth.

## Day 3

**Breakfast:** Egg and vegetable wrap.

**Instructions:** In a skillet over medium heat, heat a tablespoon of olive oil. Cook for 5 minutes after adding one cup of diced vegetables (such as bell peppers and mushrooms). Scramble two beaten eggs until they are cooked. Wrap the scramble in a tortilla and top with salsa.

**Lunch:** Salad of lentils and vegetables.

**Instructions:** Combine two cups of cooked lentils, one cup of diced vegetables (such as tomatoes and cucumbers), one tablespoon of olive oil, and one tablespoon of red wine vinegar in a large mixing bowl.

**Dinner:** Baked salmon with roasted potatoes.

**Instructions:** Preheat the oven to 375 degrees Fahrenheit. On a baking sheet, place a 6-ounce filet of salmon. Add a teaspoon of olive oil, a squeeze of lemon juice, and a pinch of salt and pepper to taste. 15 minutes in the oven. Toss one cup of diced potatoes with a teaspoon of olive oil and a pinch of salt and pepper while the salmon bakes. Bake the food on a baking pan for 20 minutes.

**Snacks:** Celery and peanut butter.

**Instructions:** Spread one tablespoon of peanut butter on each celery stick.

**Dessert:** Fruit salad.

**Instructions:** In a mixing bowl, combine 1 cup of diced strawberries, 1 cup of diced pineapple, 1 cup of diced mango, and 1 tablespoon of honey.

**Smoothie:** Banana, almond butter, and almond milk.

**Instructions:** In a blender, combine one cup of almond milk, one banana, one tablespoon of almond butter, and one tablespoon of honey. Blend until completely smooth.

## Day 4

Breakfast: Overnight oats.

**Instructions:** In a mixing bowl, combine ½ cup of rolled oats, 1 cup almond milk, 1 tablespoon of chia seeds, and 1 tablespoon of honey. Allow sitting in the refrigerator overnight. Top with a handful of berries and a tablespoon of chopped nuts in the morning.

**Lunch:** Sandwich with avocado and tomato.

**Instructions:** Spread one tablespoon of mayonnaise on two slices of whole-grain bread. One slice should be topped with ½ avocados, sliced tomato, and a pinch of salt and pepper. Top with the remaining slice of bread and cut it in half.

**Dinner:** Baked tofu with roasted vegetables.

**Instructions:** Preheat the oven to 375 degrees Fahrenheit. Cut one firm tofu block into cubes. Drizzle with olive oil and season with salt and pepper on a baking sheet. Cook for 20 minutes at 350°F. Toss one cup of chopped vegetables (such as zucchini and bell peppers) with a tablespoon of olive oil and a pinch of salt and pepper while the tofu bakes. Bake the food on a baking pan for 20 minutes.

**Snacks:** Hummus and crackers.

**Instructions:** Spread one tablespoon of hummus onto whole-grain crackers.

**Dessert:** Yogurt parfait.

**Instructions:** In a mixing bowl, combine one cup of nonfat Greek yogurt, a handful of berries, and one tablespoon of granola.

**Smoothie:** kale, banana, and almond milk.

**Instructions:** In a blender, combine one cup of almond milk, one banana, one cup of kale, and one tablespoon of honey. Blend until completely smooth.

## Day 5

**Breakfast:** Smoothie bowl.

**Instructions:** In a blender, combine one cup of almond milk, one banana, one cup of frozen blueberries, one tablespoon of almond butter, and one tablespoon of honey. Blend until completely smooth. Top with a handful of granola and a tablespoon of chopped nuts in a bowl.

**Lunch:** Burrito with quinoa and black beans.

**Instructions:** In a mixing bowl, combine 1 cup of cooked quinoa, 1 cup of cooked black beans, ½ cup of diced tomatoes, 1 tablespoon of chopped cilantro, and 1 tablespoon of lime juice. Wrap the mixture in a whole-grain tortilla.

**Dinner:** Baked chicken with roasted vegetables.

**Instructions:** Preheat the oven to 375 degrees Fahrenheit. On a baking sheet, place a 6-ounce chicken breast. Add a teaspoon of olive oil, a squeeze of lemon juice, and a pinch of salt and pepper to taste. 15 minutes in the oven. Toss one cup of chopped vegetables (such as zucchini and bell peppers) with a tablespoon of olive oil and a pinch of salt and pepper while the chicken bakes. Bake the food on a baking pan for 20 minutes.

**Snacks:** Celery and hummus.

**Instructions:** Spread one tablespoon of hummus on each celery stick.

**Dessert:** Baked apples.

**Instructions:** Preheat the oven to 375 degrees Fahrenheit. Place two apples in a baking dish and core them. Fill a tablespoon of brown sugar, one teaspoon of butter, and a sprinkle of cinnamon into the center of each apple. Cook for 20 minutes at 350°F.

**Smoothie:** Strawberries, bananas, and almond milk.

**Instructions:** In a blender, combine one cup of almond milk, one banana, one cup of frozen strawberries, and one tablespoon of honey. Blend until completely smooth.

## Day 6

**Breakfast:** Avocado toast.

**Instructions:** To begin, toast two slices of whole-grain bread. Spread 12 avocado slices on each slice and season with salt and pepper.

**Lunch:** Soup with lentils and vegetables.

**Instructions:** Sauté one diced onion, one diced bell pepper, and two cloves of minced garlic in a tablespoon of extra-virgin olive oil in a large pot over medium heat. Combine two cups of cooked lentils, four cups of vegetable broth, and one teaspoon of dried oregano in a mixing bowl. Cook for 15 minutes.

**Dinner:** Grilled fish with steamed vegetables.

**Instructions:** In a skillet over medium heat, heat a tablespoon of olive oil. Using salt and pepper, season a 6-ounce filet of fish. Cook each side for 8 minutes. Steam 1 cup of broccoli and 1 cup of cauliflower for 8 minutes while the fish is cooking.

**Snacks:** Greek yogurt and berries.

**Instructions:** Top one cup of nonfat Greek yogurt with a handful of berries.

**Dessert:** Chocolate-dipped strawberries.

**Instructions:** Melt 1 cup of dark chocolate chips in a double boiler over low heat. Place fresh strawberries on parchment paper after dipping them in melted chocolate. Cool until the chocolate has hardened.

**Smoothie:** Pineapple, banana, and almond milk.

**Instructions:** In a blender, combine one cup of almond milk, one banana, one cup of frozen pineapple, and one tablespoon of honey. Blend until completely smooth.

## Day 7

**Breakfast:** Omelet with vegetables.

**Instructions:** In a mixing bowl, whisk together two eggs. In a skillet over medium heat, heat 1 tablespoon of extra-virgin olive oil. Cook for 5 minutes after adding one cup of diced vegetables (such as bell peppers and mushrooms). Cook until the omelet is set, about 5 minutes.

**Lunch:** Quinoa and black bean salad.

**Instructions:** In a large mixing bowl, combine 2 cups cooked quinoa, 1 cup cooked black beans, ½ cup diced tomatoes, 1 tablespoon olive oil, and 1 tablespoon red wine vinegar.

**Dinner:** Baked tofu with roasted potatoes.

**Instructions:** Preheat the oven to 375 degrees Fahrenheit. Cut one firm tofu block into cubes. Drizzle with olive oil and season with salt and pepper on a baking sheet. Cook for 20 minutes at 350°F. Toss one cup of diced potatoes with a teaspoon of olive oil and a pinch of salt and pepper while the tofu bakes. Bake the food on a baking pan for 20 minutes.

**Snacks:** Apple slices with peanut butter.

**Instructions:** Spread one tablespoon of peanut butter on apple slices and serve.

**Dessert:** Yogurt parfait.

**Instructions:** In a mixing bowl, combine one cup of nonfat Greek yogurt, a handful of berries, and one tablespoon of granola.

**Smoothie:** Mango, banana, and almond milk.

**Instructions:** In a blender, combine one cup of almond milk, one banana, one cup of frozen mango, and one tablespoon of honey. Blend until completely smooth.

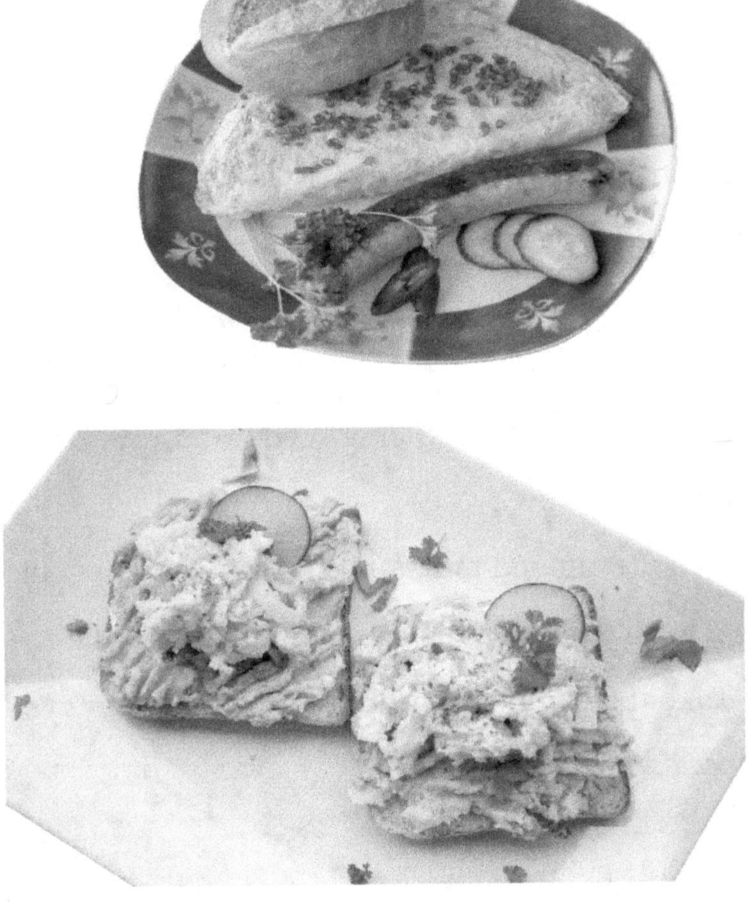

# CHAPTER 5

## 10 Cancer Diet Recipes for Newly Diagnosed:

## Breakfast

1. Chia and raisins with overnight oats (Cook Time: Overnight; Preparation Time: 5 minutes)

**Ingredients:** 1/2 cup rolled oats, 1 tablespoon chia seeds, 1 tablespoon raisins, and 1/2 cup almond milk.

**Instructions:**

- Combine the raisins, chia seeds, and rolled oats in a medium bowl.
- Add the almond milk and stir everything together.
- Place the bowl in the refrigerator for the night.
- Take the bowl out of the fridge in the morning and eat it.

2. A banana smoothie for breakfast (Prep Time: 5 minutes; Cook Time: 2 minutes)

**Ingredients:** 1 banana and 1/2 cup almond milk, 1 teaspoon chia seeds; 1 teaspoon ground flaxseed; 1 tablespoon honey

**Instructions:**

- Blend the almond milk, banana, honey, ground flaxseed, and chia seeds together in a blender.
- For 1-2 minutes, on high speed, blend the ingredients until thoroughly combined.
- Pour into a glass, then take a sip.

3. A bowl of pancakes and berries (10 minutes for preparation; 15 minutes for cooking)

**Ingredients:** 1 cup whole wheat flour, 1 tablespoon honey, 1/2 teaspoon baking soda, 1 teaspoon baking powder, 1 cup almond milk, 1 tablespoon olive oil, 1 cup mixed berries, and 1 cup plain Greek yogurt.

**Instructions:**

- Combine the flour, baking soda, baking powder, and honey in a large bowl.
- Combine the almond milk and olive oil after adding them.
- Lightly oil a skillet and heat it over medium heat.
- Using the skillet to create small pancakes, pour the batter into it.
- After cooking for 2 to 3 minutes, the pancakes should be lightly golden.
- After flipping, cook the pancakes for an additional 2 to 3 minutes.
- Arrange the pancakes in a bowl, then top them with Greek yogurt and mixed berries.

4. Egg and Spinach Baked (Prep Time: 5 minutes; Cook Time: 40 minutes)

**Ingredients:** 2 cups spinach, 4 eggs, 1 tablespoon olive oil, 1 diced onion, 2 minced garlic cloves, and 1 tablespoon olive oil

## Instructions:

- First, Set the oven to 350 degrees Fahrenheit.
- Heat the olive oil in a sizable skillet over medium heat.
- After the onion and garlic have softened, add them.
- After adding the spinach, cook it for an additional two to three minutes, or until wilted.
- Add the spinach mixture and grease a baking dish.
- Over the spinach, break the eggs, and sprinkle some salt and pepper on top.
- Bake the egg whites for 25 to 30 minutes, or until they are fully set.
- Take out of the oven and savor.

5. Toast with sweet potato (Prep Time: 5 minutes; Cook Time: 10 minutes)

**Ingredients:** 1 sweet potato, 2 tablespoons of almond butter, 1 teaspoon each of honey and ground cinnamon, and 1 tablespoon of chia seeds.

**Instructions:**

- Set the oven to 375 degrees.

- Cut the sweet potato into slices that are 1/4 inch thick.

- Arrange the sweet potato slices on a baking sheet and bake for 10 minutes, turning once.

- Remove from the oven and sprinkle with cinnamon, honey, chia seeds, and almond butter.

6. Cheese and broccoli in an omelet (10 minutes for preparation; 10 minutes for cooking)

**Ingredients:** 2 eggs, 2 tablespoons milk, 1/2 cup chopped broccoli, 2 tablespoons shredded cheddar cheese, and 1 tablespoon extra virgin olive oil. To taste, add salt and pepper

**Instructions:**

- In a medium mixing bowl, combine the milk and eggs.

- In a skillet over medium heat, warm the olive oil.

- After adding it, cook the broccoli for 4–5 minutes, or until it softens.

- Add the egg mixture and add salt and pepper to taste.

- Cook the eggs for 2 to 3 minutes, or until they are barely set.

- Top the omelet with cheddar cheese and fold it in half.

- Continue cooking for a further 1-2 minutes, or until the cheese is melted.

- Discard the heat and savor.

7. Tomato and avocado toast (5 minutes for preparation; 0 minutes for cooking)

**Ingredients:** two slices of whole wheat bread, one tomato, two tablespoons of feta cheese, one half of an avocado, mashed.

**Instructions:**

- Bread should be toasted until golden.

- Cover the toast with the mashed avocado.

- Add feta cheese and tomato slices on top.

- Add salt and pepper to taste.

8. Muffins with egg and cheese (Prep Time: 10 minutes; Cook Time: 20 minutes)

**Ingredients:** ½ cup shredded cheddar cheese, 2 tablespoons chopped scallions, 2 eggs, 2 tablespoons milk, ½ cup whole wheat flour, and 1/2 teaspoon baking powder, To taste add salt and pepper.

**Instructions:**

- Set the oven to 375 degrees.

- Use oil to grease a muffin pan.

- In a medium mixing bowl, combine the milk and eggs.

- Add the cheddar cheese and scallions after that.

- Combine the flour, baking powder, salt, and pepper in a different bowl.

- Add the flour mixture and stir it into the egg mixture.
- Place the muffin tin with the batter in it, and bake for 20 minutes, or until golden.
- Enjoy.

9. Salsa-topped breakfast burrito (Prep Time: 10 minutes; Cook Time: 10 minutes)

**Ingredients:** two eggs, two tablespoons of salsa, two tablespoons of shredded cheddar cheese, two tablespoons of black beans, two tablespoons of diced bell pepper, two tablespoons of diced onion, two tortillas made from whole wheat, and salt and pepper to taste.

**Instructions:**

- Lightly oil a skillet and heat it over medium heat.
- After cracking the eggs, add salt and pepper to the skillet.
- Cook the eggs for two to three minutes while stirring occasionally.

- Stir in the salsa, cheddar cheese, black beans, bell pepper, and onion after taking the eggs off the heat.

- Arrange a tortilla on a plate and top it with the egg mixture.

- Place the second tortilla on top, then fold it over the filling.

- If desired, serve with extra salsa.

10. Fruit and Granola Yogurt Parfait (10 minutes for preparation; 0 minutes for cooking)

**Ingredients:** ½ cup granola, ½ cup plain Greek yogurt, and ½ cup mixed berries.

**Instructions:**

- Arrange the yogurt, granola, and berries in a bowl or glass.

# Lunch

1. Chickpea salad from the Mediterranean (Prep Time: 10 minutes)

**Ingredients:**

-1 can (14.5 ounces) chickpeas, drained and rinsed

-1/3 cup fresh parsley leaves, chopped

-1/2 cup red onion, diced

-1/2 cup cucumber, diced

-1/2 cup grape tomatoes, halved

-1/4 cup Kalamata olives, halved

-1/4 cup olive oil

-2 tablespoons red wine vinegar

-1 teaspoon garlic, minced

-1/2 teaspoon dried oregano

-1/4 teaspoon sea salt

**Instructions:**

- Combine the chickpeas, parsley, red onion, cucumber, tomatoes, and olives in a medium bowl.
- Combine the olive oil, red wine vinegar, garlic, oregano, and sea salt in a small bowl.
- After adding the dressing, combine the chickpea mixture by gently stirring.
- Whether at room temperature or chilled, serve.

2. Veggie bowl with roasting (Prep Time: 25 minutes)

**Ingredients:**

-one small sweet potato, diced; one red bell pepper, diced; and half a red onion, diced.

-broccoli florets, 1 cup

-Cauliflower florets, 1 cup

-Olive oil, two tablespoons

-one-fourth teaspoon sea salt and one-fourth teaspoon black pepper

-One-fourth teaspoon of garlic powder

**Instructions:**

- Set the oven to 400 degrees.
- Arrange the sweet potato, red onion, bell pepper, broccoli, and cauliflower on a sizable baking sheet. Sprinkle with sea salt, black pepper, and garlic powder after drizzling with olive oil.
- Roast the vegetables in the preheated oven for 20 to 25 minutes, or until they are soft and just beginning to brown.
- Present hot.

3. Salmon baked with vegetables (25 minutes for preparation)

**Ingredients:** Salmon fillet, one pound, one tablespoon olive oil, one-fourth teaspoon sea salt, and one-fourth teaspoon black pepper, 1 cup chopped asparagus, 1 cup halved cherry tomatoes, 1/2 cup diced red onion, and 1/4 cup chopped fresh parsley.

**Instructions:**

- Set the oven to 375 degrees.
- On a sizable baking sheet, arrange the salmon fillet. Add the sea salt and black pepper, then drizzle with the olive oil.
- Place the salmon in the center of the asparagus, tomatoes, and red onion.
- Bake for 20 to 25 minutes in a preheated oven, or until the salmon is cooked through and the vegetables are soft.
- Just before serving, garnish with fresh parsley.

4. Mexican-style vegan quinoa bowl (Prep Time: 15 minutes)

**Ingredients:** 1 cup of rinsed and drained black beans and 1 can (15 ounces) of quinoa, 1 cup of frozen or canned corn, 1/2 cup of diced red bell pepper. 1/2 cup diced red onion, 1/2 cup halved cherry tomatoes, 1/4 cup chopped fresh cilantro, two tablespoons each of lime juice and olive oil, one teaspoon of chili powder, 1-fourth teaspoon of sea salt.

**Instructions:**

- Cook the quinoa according to the package directions.
- Combine the prepared quinoa, black beans, corn, bell pepper, red onion, tomatoes, and cilantro in a sizable bowl.
- Combine the olive oil, lime juice, chili powder, and sea salt in a small bowl.
- After adding the dressing, add the quinoa mixture and gently mix everything together.
- Whether at room temperature or chilled, serve.

5. Vegetable lentil soup (Prep Time: 15 minutes)

**Ingredients:** 1 tablespoon olive oil, 1 diced onion, 2 minced garlic cloves, 1 diced carrot, 1 diced celery stalk, 1 can (14.5 ounces) of diced tomatoes, 2 cups of vegetable broth, and 1 cup of lentils, half a teaspoon of dried oregano, one-fourth teaspoon sea salt and one-fourth teaspoon black pepper.

**Instructions:**

- Warm the olive oil in a skillet over medium heat.
- After the onion has softened, add the garlic and cook for an additional 3 to 4 minutes.
- Include the celery and carrot and cook for an additional 3 to 4 minutes.
- Add the tomato, lentil, oregano, sea salt, and black pepper to the vegetable broth. Bring to a boil, then lower the heat and simmer the lentils for 10 to 15 minutes, or until they are tender.
- Present hot.

6. Apples and cranberries with kale salad (Prep Time: 10 minutes)

**Ingredients:** 1 bunch chopped kale, 1/2 cup diced apples, 1/4 cup dried cranberries, Olive oil two tablespoons, 1/4 teaspoon sea salt, 2 tablespoons apple cider vinegar, and 1/4 teaspoon black pepper.

**Instructions:**

- Combine the kale, apples, and cranberries in a big bowl.

- Combine the olive oil, apple cider vinegar, sea salt, and black pepper in a small bowl.

- Drizzle the dressing over the kale mixture and toss everything together gently.

- Serve at room temperature or chilled.

7. Roasted vegetables with zucchini noodles (25 minutes for preparation)

**Ingredients:** 3 zucchinis, spiralized, 1 red bell pepper, diced, 1/2 red onion, diced, 1 cup mushrooms sliced, and 2 tablespoons olive oil.

**Instructions:**

- Set the oven to 400 degrees.

- Arrange the bell pepper, red onion, and mushrooms on a sizable baking sheet. Add the sea salt and black pepper, then drizzle with the olive oil.

- Roast the vegetables in the preheated oven for 20 to 25 minutes, or until they are soft and just beginning to brown.
- Combine the roasted vegetables and spiralized zucchini noodles in a big bowl.
- Present hot.

8. Quinoa and Avocado Salad (Prep Time: 10 minutes)

**Ingredients:**

-1 cup cooked quinoa, 1 diced avocado, and 1/2 cup diced cucumber

-1/4 cup diced red onion

-1/4 cup chopped sun-dried tomatoes

-two tablespoons each of lemon juice and olive oil

-one-fourth teaspoon sea salt and one-fourth teaspoon black pepper

**Instructions:**

- Place the cooked quinoa, avocado, cucumber, red onion, and sun-dried tomatoes in a large bowl.
- Combine the olive oil, lemon juice, sea salt, and black pepper in a small bowl.
- Drizzle the dressing over the quinoa mixture, then toss everything together gently.
- Whether at room temperature or chilled, serve.

9. Vegetable and Hummus Wrap (Prep Time: 10 minutes)

**Ingredients:** two whole wheat tortillas, one-fourth cup of hummus, half a cup of grated carrots, 1/2 cup sliced cucumber, 1/4 cup diced red onion.

**Instructions:**

- Spread the hummus on the tortillas
- Add the red onion, cucumber, and carrots on top.
- Cut the tortillas in half after rolling them up.
- Whether at room temperature or chilled, serve.

10. Avocado and Egg Salad (Prep Time: 10 minutes)

**Ingredients:**

-4 hard-boiled eggs, peeled and chopped

-1 avocado, diced

-1/2 cup celery, diced

-2 tablespoons plain Greek yogurt

-2 tablespoons mayonnaise

-1 teaspoon mustard

-1/4 teaspoon sea salt

-1/4 teaspoon black pepper

**Instructions:**

- Combine the celery, avocado, and hard-boiled eggs in a big bowl.
- Combine the yogurt, mayonnaise, mustard, sea salt, and black pepper in a small bowl.

- After adding the dressing to the egg mixture, gently fold everything together.

- Whether at room temperature or chilled, serve.

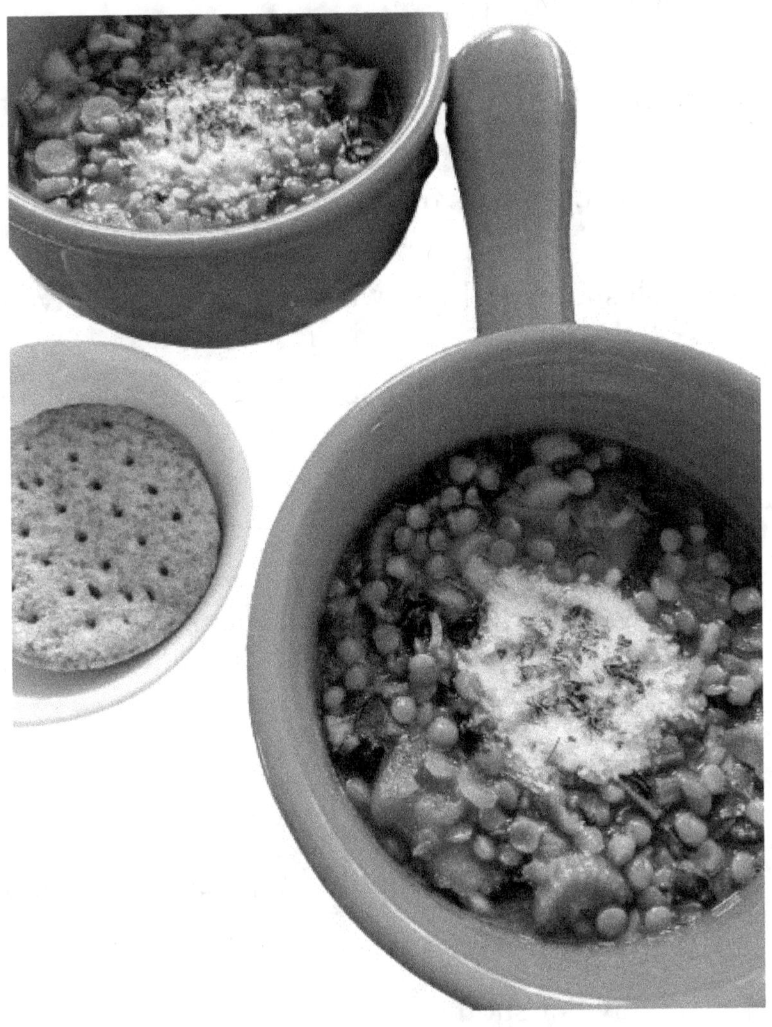

# Dinner

1. Baked salmon with sweet potatoes and broccoli (45 minutes, serves 4)

## Ingredients:

- 4 (4-ounce) fillets of salmon

- 1 tablespoon garlic powder - 2 teaspoons olive oil

- 2 cups of cut-up broccoli; - 1/2 teaspoon of ground black pepper; - 1/4 teaspoon of sea salt

- 2 cups peeled and chopped into 1-inch cubes sweet potatoes - 2 teaspoons freshly squeezed lemon juice

## Instructions:

- Set the oven to 400 degrees.
- Salmon fillets should be placed in a small baking dish and brushed with oil. Salt, pepper, and garlic powder should be added.

- Set the salmon in the center of the broccoli and sweet potatoes. Add a lemon juice drizzle.
- 25 minutes in the oven. Serve hot.

2. Peppers with quinoa and vegetables inside (55 minutes, serves 4)

**Ingredients:**

- 4 peppers of any color, bell

-Olive oil, 1 tablespoon

- 1/2 cup diced red onion

- 1 cup diced mushrooms

- 1 minced garlic clove

-1 tsp. dried oregano

-1/2 teaspoon each of ground cumin and ground black pepper

- One-fourth teaspoon of sea salt

- 1 serving of cooked quinoa

- 1/2 cup corn and 1 cup black beans, cooked

- Half a cup of cherry tomatoes

## Instructions:

- Set the oven to 375 degrees.
- Cut the bell peppers' tops off and scoop out the seeds and membranes. Peppers should be put in a baking pan.
- Add onion, mushrooms, garlic, oregano, cumin, pepper, and salt to a large skillet of olive oil that has been heated to medium-high heat. While occasionally stirring, cook for 5 minutes.
- Include tomatoes, corn, black beans, and quinoa. Cook for a further five minutes.
- Place the peppers with the quinoa mixture inside. Bake for 30 minutes with the foil covering the baking dish. Serve hot.

3. Vegetables and Chicken Roasted (60 min., 4 servings)

**Ingredients:**

- 4 skinless, boneless breasts of chicken

- 1 tablespoon garlic powder - 2 teaspoons olive oil

- 1/2 teaspoon oregano, dried

-1/2 teaspoon each of ground cumin and ground black pepper

- One-fourth teaspoon of sea salt

- 2 cups each of broccoli and cauliflower florets

- 2 cups peeled and chopped into 1-inch cubes of sweet potatoes

 - 2 teaspoons freshly squeezed lemon juice

**Instructions:**

- Set the oven to 400 degrees.

- Spread oil over the chicken breasts and place them in a small baking dish. Add salt, pepper, oregano, cumin, and garlic powder.

- Position the sweet potatoes, broccoli, and cauliflower around the chicken. Add a lemon juice drizzle.

- 25 minutes in the oven. Serve hot.

4. Brown rice and salmon that has been grilled (45 minutes, serves 4)

**Ingredients:**

- 4 salmon fillets, each weighing 4 ounces; - 2 tablespoons olive oil; - 1 teaspoon garlic powder

- Add half a teaspoon of black pepper, ground

- One-fourth teaspoon of sea salt

- 1 pound of trimmed asparagus

-2 cups of cooked brown rice

- Freshly squeezed lemon juice, 2 tablespoons

**Instructions:**

- Turn the grill's heat up to medium-high.
- Salmon fillets should be placed in a shallow dish and brushed with oil. Salt, pepper, and garlic powder should be added.
- For five minutes, grill the asparagus.
- Grill the salmon on both sides for 4 minutes.
- Include brown rice and asparagus with the salmon on the menu. Add a lemon juice drizzle.

5. Stir-Fry with Baked Tofu and Vegetables (50 minutes, serves 4)

**Ingredients:**

-1 (14-ounce) package of cubed, extra-firm tofu, 2 tablespoons of olive oil, and 1 teaspoon of garlic powder.

- Add half a teaspoon of black pepper, ground

- One-fourth teaspoon of sea salt

-2-cups of broccoli florets

- 2 cups florets of cauliflower

- 2 cups sliced mushrooms

- 2 cups sliced red bell pepper

-2 tablespoons of orange juice that has just been squeezed

**Instructions:**

- Set the oven to 400 degrees.

- Spread some oil in a shallow baking dish and add the tofu cubes. Salt, pepper, and garlic powder should be added.

- Place the bell pepper, bell mushroom, broccoli, and cauliflower around the tofu. Orange juice should be drizzled.

- 25 minutes in the oven. Serve hot.

6. Baked cod with tomatoes and zucchini (45 minutes, serves 4)

## Ingredients:

- 4 cod fillets, each weighing 4 ounces

- 2 tablespoons olive oil

- 1 teaspoon garlic powder

- Add half a teaspoon of black pepper, ground

- One-fourth teaspoon of sea salt

- 2 cups sliced zucchini

- 2 cups halved cherry tomatoes

- 2 tablespoons lemon juice

## Instructions:

- Set the oven to 400 degrees.

- Cod fillets should be placed in a shallow baking dish and brushed with oil. Salt, pepper, and garlic powder should be added.
- Position the tomatoes and zucchini around the cod. Add a lemon juice drizzle.
- 25 minutes in the oven. Serve hot.

7. Baked vegetables and tempeh (4 serves, 45 minutes)

**Ingredients:**

-Cubed tempeh from a single 8-ounce package, 2 tablespoons of olive oil, and 1 teaspoon of garlic powder

- Add half a teaspoon of black pepper, ground

- One-fourth teaspoon of sea salt

- 2 cups halved Brussels sprouts

- 2 cups peeled and sliced carrots

- 2 tablespoons lime juice that has just been squeezed

## Instructions:

- Set the oven to 400 degrees.
- Spread some oil in a shallow baking dish and add the tempeh cubes. Salt, pepper, and garlic powder should be added.
- Position the tempeh around the carrots and Brussels sprouts. Add lime juice as a drizzle.
- 25 minutes in the oven. Serve hot.

8. Baked Fish with Spinach and Potatoes (45 minutes, serves 4)

## Ingredients:

- 4 white fish fillets, each weighing 4 ounces;

- 2 tablespoons olive oil; - 1 teaspoon garlic powder

- Add half a teaspoon of black pepper, ground

- One-fourth teaspoon of sea salt

- 2 cups peeled and chopped into 1-inch cubes of potatoes

- 2 cups spinach - 2 tablespoons lemon juice that has just been squeezed

**Instructions:**

- Set the oven to 400 degrees.
- Arrange the fish fillets in a baking dish that is not too deep and brush them with oil. Salt, pepper, and garlic powder should be added.
- Position the fish in the center of the potatoes and spinach. Add a lemon juice drizzle.
- 25 minutes in the oven. Serve hot.

9. Bowl with Broccoli and Baked Tofu (45 minutes, serves 4)

**Ingredients:**

-1 (14-ounce) package of cubed, extra-firm tofu, 2 tablespoons of olive oil, and 1 teaspoon of garlic powder.

- Add half a teaspoon of black pepper, ground

- Two cups broccoli florets - One-fourth teaspoon of sea salt

-2 tablespoons of orange juice that has just been squeezed

-2 cups of cooked brown rice

**Instructions:**

- Set the oven to 400 degrees.
- Spread some oil in a shallow baking dish and add the tofu cubes. Salt, pepper, and garlic powder should be added.
- Put the broccoli in a circle around the tofu. Orange juice should be drizzled.
- 25 minutes in the oven.
- Spread a bed of brown rice with the baked tofu.

10. Sweet potatoes and green beans with baked chicken (4 serves, 45 minutes)

**Ingredients:**

- 4 skinless, boneless breasts of chicken

- 1 tablespoon garlic powder - 2 teaspoons olive oil

- Add half a teaspoon of black pepper, ground

- 2 cups sweet potatoes, peeled and cut into 1-inch cubes

- 1/4 teaspoon sea salt

- 2 cups green beans

- 2 tablespoons lemon juice that has just been squeezed

**Instructions:**

- Set the oven to 400 degrees.
- Spread oil over the chicken breasts and place them in a small baking dish. Salt, pepper, and garlic powder should be added.
- Position the chicken around the sweet potatoes and green beans. Add a lemon juice drizzle.
- 25 minutes in the oven. Serve hot.

1. Cookie bites with chocolate, banana, and oats

For cancer patients who have just received a diagnosis, these chocolate banana oatmeal cookie bites make a quick and wholesome snack. This snack will undoubtedly provide energy and nutrition to those who need it most because it is stuffed with fiber, protein, and antioxidants.

**Ingredients:**

-Contains one banana.

- Cocoa powder, 2 tablespoons

- Peanut butter, 2 tablespoons

-Old-fashioned oats in a cup with a teaspoon of honey

**Instructions:**

- Set the oven's temperature to 350 F.
- In a medium bowl, mash the banana until it is creamy.

- Include honey, oats, peanut butter, cocoa powder, and honey. Combine each ingredient in the mixture.
- Line a baking sheet with parchment paper.
- Make small balls out of the cookie dough and set them on the baking sheet.
- Bake for 15 minutes, until the top, is golden brown.
- Allow to cool and delight!

Prep Time: 15 minutes

2. Fries made of sweet potatoes

An excellent and healthy snack for cancer patients who have just been diagnosed is sweet potato fries. Sweet potatoes are a great snack for people trying to get their recommended daily intake of nutrition because they are high in fiber, vitamins, and minerals.

**Ingredients:**

-1 teaspoon of garlic powder

- 2 large sweet potatoes

-2 tablespoons of olive oil

- One teaspoon of onion powder

-Smoked paprika, 1 teaspoon

-salt, 1 teaspoon

## Instructions:

- Set the oven's temperature to 400 F.
- Make thin fries out of sweet potatoes.
- Add the olive oil, smoked paprika, garlic powder, onion powder, and salt to the large bowl of fries. Fries should be coated evenly after being tossed.
- Line a baking sheet with parchment paper.
- Arrange the fries evenly across the baking sheet.
- Bake for 30 minutes, or until the pastry is crisp and golden brown.
- Allow to cool and delight!

Prep Time: 40 minutes

3. Roasted chickpeas

An excellent snack for cancer patients who have just received a diagnosis is roasted chickpeas. This snack is a great way to get the nutrition you require because it is packed with fiber, protein, and important vitamins and minerals.

**Ingredients:**

-chickpeas, one can

- 1 tablespoon garlic powder

- One teaspoon of onion powder

-Smoked paprika 1 teaspoon

-salt 1 teaspoon

**Instructions:**

- Set the oven's temperature to 375 F.
- Rinse and drain the chickpeas.

- Add the salt, smoked paprika, olive oil, garlic powder, onion powder, and chickpeas to a large bowl. Make sure the chickpeas are evenly coated by tossing them.
- Line a baking sheet with parchment paper.
- Scatter the chickpeas evenly across the baking sheet.
- Bake for 30 minutes, or until the pastry is crisp and golden brown.
- Allow to cool and delight!

Prep Time: 40 minutes

4. Spinach and artichoke dip

An excellent snack for cancer patients who have just received a diagnosis is spinach artichoke dip. This dip, which is rich in vitamins and minerals, will give you the energy and nutrition you need to fight cancer.

**Ingredients:**

- 1 cup of thawed and drained frozen spinach - 1 can of drained artichoke hearts - 1 cup of plain Greek yogurt

- 1 tablespoon garlic powder - 2 teaspoons olive oil

- One teaspoon of onion powder

- 1/2 tsp. smoked paprika

**Instructions:**

- Set the oven's temperature to 350 F.
- Combine the spinach, artichoke hearts, Greek yogurt, olive oil, garlic powder, onion powder, and smoked paprika in a medium bowl.
- Use parchment paper to line a baking pan.
- Evenly distribute the dip throughout the baking dish.
- Bake for 15 minutes, or until the top is golden.
- Allow to cool and delight!

Prep Time: 25 minutes

5. Vegetable Medley, Roasted

For cancer patients who have just received a diagnosis, a delicious and nourishing snack is a roasted vegetable medley. This snack, which is rich in vitamins and minerals, will provide them with the nutrition and energy they require.

**Ingredients:**

- 2 cups of finely chopped vegetables (any combination of carrots, bell peppers, onions, mushrooms, asparagus, etc.)

- 1 tablespoon garlic powder - 2 teaspoons olive oil

- One teaspoon of onion powder

-Smoked paprika, 1 teaspoon

-salt, 1 teaspoon

**Instructions:**

- Set the oven's temperature to 400 F.

- Add the salt, smoked paprika, olive oil, garlic powder, onion powder, and chopped vegetables to a large bowl. The vegetables should be coated evenly after being tossed.
- Line a baking sheet with parchment paper.
- Arrange the vegetables evenly on the baking sheet.
- Bake for 25 minutes, until tender and golden brown.
- Allow to cool and delight!

Prep Time: 30 minutes

6. Baked Apples

An excellent snack for cancer patients who have just received a diagnosis is baked apples. This snack will provide them with the energy and nutrition they require because it is rich in fiber and nutrients.

**Ingredients:**

-Two apples

- 1 teaspoon of cinnamon

- One tablespoon of honey

**Instructions:**

- Set the oven's temperature to 350 F.
- Slice the apples.
- Add the honey, cinnamon, and coconut oil to the medium bowl with the apple slices. The apples should be evenly coated after being tossed.
- Line a baking sheet with parchment paper.
- Arrange the apples evenly across the baking sheet.
- Bake for twenty minutes, until tender and golden brown.
- Allow to cool and delight!

Prep Time: 25 minutes

7. Energy Bites with peanut butter and jelly

For cancer patients who have recently received a diagnosis, peanut butter, and jelly energy bites make a great snack. This snack will provide them with the necessary nutrition and energy because it is packed with fiber, protein, and important vitamins and minerals.

**Ingredients:**

-Old-fashioned oats, 1 cup

-peanut butter, 1/2 cup

- 1 cup of raisins

-honey, 2 tablespoons

**Instructions:**

- Fill a big bowl with oats.
- Include honey, dried fruit, and peanut butter. Combine each ingredient in the mixture.
- Make little balls out of the mixture and put them in an airtight container.
- Put the food in the fridge at least an hour before serving.
- Enjoy!

Prep Time: 10 minutes

## 8. Trail Mix

For cancer patients who have recently received a diagnosis, trail mix is a great snack. This snack will provide them with the necessary nutrition and energy because it is loaded with fiber, protein, and important vitamins and minerals.

**Ingredients:**

-almonds, 1 cup

-walnuts, 1 cup

- 1/2 cup dried cranberries

- 1/2 cup dried cherries

**Instructions:**

- In a medium bowl, combine the almonds, walnuts, dried cranberries, and dried cherries.
- Combine all the ingredients by combining them thoroughly.
- Keep the container airtight.

Prep Time: 5 minutes

## 9. Apple and Walnut Salad

An excellent snack for cancer patients who have just received a diagnosis is apple and walnut salad. This snack will provide them with the necessary nutrition and energy because it is packed with fiber, protein, and important vitamins and minerals.

**Ingredients:**

- 2 diced apples

-1/2 cup chopped walnuts

- 2 tablespoons extra virgin olive oil

- 1 teaspoon honey

- 2 diced apples

**Instructions:**

- Fill a medium bowl with the chopped walnuts and diced apples.

- Include lemon juice, honey, and olive oil. The ingredients should be coated evenly after being tossed.

- Put the food in the fridge at least an hour before serving.

Prep Time: 10 minutes

10. Avocado Toast

A great snack for cancer patients who have just received a diagnosis is avocado toast. This snack will provide them with the nutrition and energy they require because it is packed with good fats, vitamins, and minerals.

**Ingredients:**

- 2 slices of whole wheat bread

- 1 avocado, mashed

- 2 tablespoons olive oil

- 1 tablespoon garlic powder

## Instructions:

- The bread should be toasted until golden brown.
- Evenly spread mashed avocado on each piece of toast.
- Sprinkle each piece of toast with a little salt, garlic powder, and olive oil.

Prep Time: 5 minutes

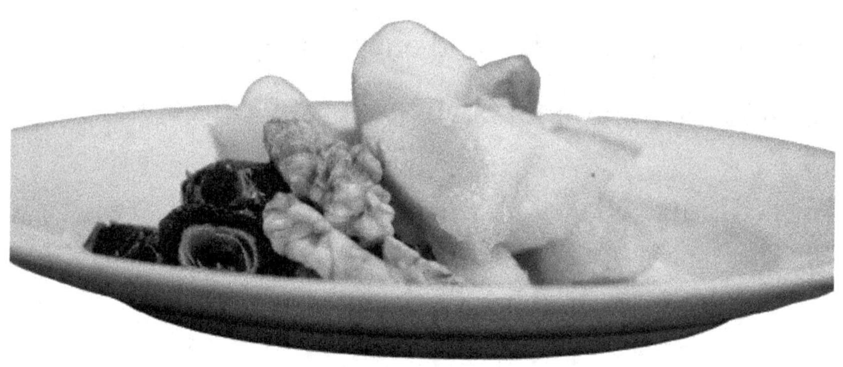

Newly diagnosed cancer patients will love these 10 delectable and healthy dessert recipes. They can give you a healthy boost of antioxidants and other necessary nutrients, and they're simple to make. All of the recipes are simple to modify to adhere to dietary restrictions and are low in sugar and fat.

1. Banana Walnut Muffins

**Ingredients:**

-2 cups all-purpose flour

- One teaspoon of baking soda

- 1/4 cup olive oil

- 1/2 teaspoon salt

– 1/4 cup honey

- 2 eggs

- Two mashed bananas

\- 1/4 cup walnuts, chopped

## Instructions:

- Set the oven to 350 degrees.

- In a medium mixing basin, combine the flour, baking soda, baking powder, and salt.

- Combine olive oil, honey, eggs, and banana in a different bowl.

- Combine the dry ingredients just before adding the wet ingredients.

- Stir in the walnuts.

- Grease a 12-cup muffin tin and fill each one with batter to about 3/4 full.

- Bake the cake for 20 minutes, or until a toothpick inserted in the middle comes out clean.

Prep time: 15 minutes

2. Bars made with apple and cinnamon

**Ingredients:**

2 cups old-fashioned oats, 1/2 cup almond flour, 1/2 cup brown sugar, and 2 teaspoons of ground cinnamon are the ingredients.

3 tablespoons of honey, ¼ teaspoon of salt, and ½ cup of melted coconut oil, and 2 diced and peeled apples.

**Instructions:**

- Set the oven to 350 degrees.
- Combine the oats, almond flour, brown sugar, cinnamon, and salt in a medium bowl.
- Combine the dry ingredients by stirring in the honey and melted coconut oil.
- Fill the bottom of an 8x8-inch baking pan with the oat mixture.
- Scatter the apple dice over the oat mixture.
- Bake for 25 minutes, or until the top is golden.

Prep time: 10 minutes

3. Chocolate Avocado Pudding

**Ingredients:**

- 2 ripe avocados

- ½ cup cocoa powder

- ¼ cup honey

- 2 tablespoons almond milk

- ½ teaspoon vanilla extract

**Instructions:**

- Blend avocados, cocoa powder, honey, almond milk, and vanilla extract in a food processor.
- Process just until creamy and smooth.
- Separate the pudding into 4 tiny bowls.
- Before serving, place in the fridge for at least an hour.

Prep time: 10 minutes

4. Berry No-Bake Cheesecake

**Ingredients:**

-One cup of Graham Cracker Crumbs

- 2 packages of softened 8-ounce cream cheese

- 1 teaspoon vanilla extract

- 2 cups of fresh berries

- 3/4 cup of honey

- 2 cups of fresh berries

**Instructions:**

- Combine melted coconut oil and graham cracker crumbs in a medium bowl.
- Press into an 8-inch springform pan's bottom.
- Combine cream cheese, honey, and vanilla extract in a big bowl and beat until fluffy.
- Cover the graham cracker crust with the cream cheese mixture.

- Add fresh berries on top.
- Before serving, place in the refrigerator for at least two hours.

Prep time: 15 minutes

5. Yogurt Berry Parfait

**Ingredients:**

- 1 cup plain Greek yogurt

- 1 tablespoon honey

- ½ teaspoon ground cinnamon

- 2 cups fresh or frozen berries

**Instructions:**

- Combine yogurt, honey, and cinnamon in a small bowl.
- Arrange berries and yogurt mixture in a tall glass or parfait dish.

- Before serving, place in the fridge for at least 30 minutes.

Prep time: 10 minutes

6. Chocolate Peanut Butter No-Bake Bars

**Ingredients:**

- 2 cups rolled oats

- ½ cup peanut butter

- ½ cup honey

- ½ cup cocoa powder

**Instructions:**

- Combine the oats, peanut butter, honey, and cocoa powder in a medium bowl.
- Combine thoroughly by mixing.
- Butter an 8x8-inch baking dish.
- Firmly press the oat mixture into the pan's bottom.
- Before slicing, refrigerate for at least an hour.

Prep time: 10 minutes

7. Carrot cake

**Ingredients:**

-2-cups of all-purpose flour

- 1 teaspoon each of baking soda and baking powder

- 1 teaspoon cinnamon, ground

- 1/4 cup olive oil

- 1/2 cup honey

- ½ teaspoon salt

- 2 eggs

-2 cups of grated carrots

- 1/4 cup walnuts, chopped

**Instructions:**

- Set the oven to 350 degrees.
- Combine the flour, baking soda, baking powder, cinnamon, and salt in a medium bowl.

- Combine the olive oil, honey, eggs, and carrots in a different bowl.
- Combine the dry ingredients just before adding the wet ingredients.
- Stir in the walnuts.
- Add batter to a greased 9-inch cake pan.
- Bake the cake for 30 minutes, or until a toothpick inserted in the middle comes out clean.

Prep time: 15 minutes

8. Orange Almond Cake

**Ingredients:**

- 2 cups all-purpose flour

- 1 teaspoon baking soda

- One teaspoon of baking soda

- 1/4 cup olive oil

- 1/2 teaspoon salt

– 1/4 cup honey

- 2 eggs

- 2 tablespoons orange zest

- 1/4 cup chopped almonds

## Instructions:

- Set the oven to 350 degrees.
- In a medium mixing basin, combine the flour, baking soda, baking powder, and salt.
- Combine olive oil, honey, eggs, and orange zest in a different bowl.
- Combine the dry ingredients just before adding the wet ingredients.
- Combine almonds.
- Add batter to a greased 9-inch cake pan.
- Bake the cake for 30 minutes, or until a toothpick inserted in the middle comes out clean.

Prep time: 15 minutes

## 9. Bake-Free Coconut Macaroons

**Ingredients:** two cups of coconut flakes, one-half cup of honey, two tablespoons of coconut oil, and two tablespoons of almond milk.

**Instructions:**

- Combine the shredded coconut, honey, coconut oil, and almond milk in a medium bowl.
- Combine thoroughly by mixing.
- Oil a baking pan.
- Spoon heaping tablespoons of the coconut mixture onto the baking sheet.
- Put the food in the fridge at least an hour before serving.

Prep time: 10 minutes

## 10. Cups of chocolate and peanut butter

**Ingredients:** 2 tablespoons of honey, 1/2 cup of peanut butter, 1/4 cup cacao powder, One-fourth cup of melted coconut oil

**Instructions:**

- Combine peanut butter, honey, and cocoa powder in a small bowl.
- Fill each cup of a mini muffin tin with one tablespoon of the peanut butter mixture.
- Drizzle the top with melted coconut oil.
- Put the food in the fridge at least an hour before serving.

Prep time: 10 minutes

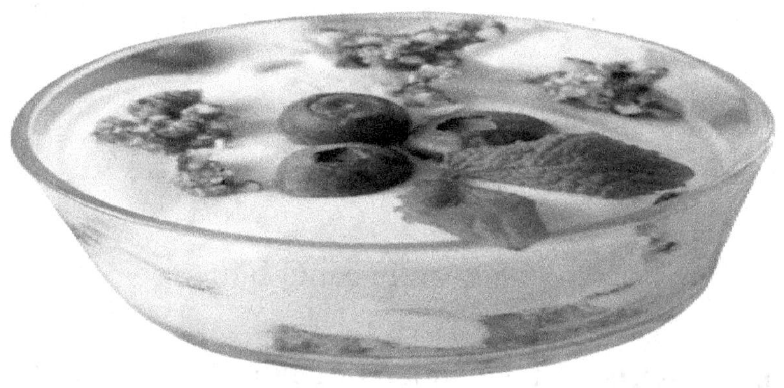

# Smoothies

These ten smoothie recipes were created especially for people who have just received a cancer diagnosis. These recipes are all delicious, simple to prepare, and packed with nutrients.

1. Smoothie with blueberries and bananas

**Ingredients:**

A single frozen banana

1 cup of blueberries, frozen

A single cup of almond milk

A single scoop of vegan protein powder

Honey, one tablespoon

**Instructions:**

- All the components should be put in a blender.
- Blend until smooth.

Prep Time: 5 minutes

2. A carrot-beet smoothie

**Ingredients:**

A single frozen banana

12 cups of cooked beets

half a cup of cooked carrots

1 cup of almond milk without sugar

A single scoop of vegan protein powder

Honey, one tablespoon

**Instructions:**

- All the components should be put in a blender.
- Blend until smooth.

Prep Time: 5 minutes

3. A kale and avocado smoothie

**Ingredients:**

A single frozen banana

Half a cup of kale

A half avocado

1 cup of almond milk without sugar

A single scoop of vegan protein powder

Honey, one tablespoon

**Instructions:**

- All the components should be put in a blender.
- Blend until smooth.

Prep Time: 5 minutes

4. A spinach and mango smoothie

**Ingredients:**

A single frozen banana

1/2 cup of frozen mango

1/2 cup of spinach

1 cup of almond milk without sugar

A single scoop of vegan protein powder

Honey, one tablespoon

**Instructions:**

- All the components should be put in a blender.
- Blend until smooth.

Prep Time: 5 minutes

5. Smoothie with strawberry and coconut

**Ingredients:**

A single frozen banana

1 cup of strawberries, frozen

1/4 cup of coconut flakes without sugar

1 cup of almond milk without sugar

A single scoop of vegan protein powder

Honey, one tablespoon

**Instructions:**

- All the components should be put in a blender.
- Blend until smooth.

Prep Time: 5 minutes

6. Apple-Cinnamon Smoothie

**Ingredients:**

A single frozen banana

1/2 cup of apple dice

Cinnamon, 1 teaspoon

1 cup of almond milk without sugar

A single scoop of vegan protein powder

Honey, one tablespoon

**Instructions:**

- All the components should be put in a blender.
- Purée until fluid.

Prep Time: 5 minutes

7. Pineapple-Ginger Smoothie

**Ingredients:**

A single frozen banana

1/2 cup of pineapple, frozen

1 cup of unsweetened almond milk and 1 teaspoon of freshly grated ginger

A single scoop of vegan protein powder

Honey, one tablespoon

**Instructions:**

- All the components should be put in a blender.
- Purée until fluid.

Prep Time: 5 minutes

8. Acai Berry Smoothie

**Ingredients:**

A single frozen banana

Acai berry powder, 1/4 cup

1/4 cup of berries, frozen

1 cup of almond milk without sugar

A single scoop of vegan protein powder

Honey, one tablespoon

**Instructions:**

- All the components should be put in a blender.
- Purée until fluid.

Prep Time: 5 minutes

9. Cherry Chia Smoothie

**Ingredients:**

A single frozen banana

Chia seeds, 1/4 cup

Frozen cherries, 1/4 cup

1 cup of almond milk without sugar

A single scoop of vegan protein powder

Honey, one tablespoon

**Instructions:**

- All the components should be put in a blender.
- Purée until fluid.

Prep Time: 5 minutes

10. Ginger-Pumpkin Smoothie

Ingredients:

1 frozen banana

1/4 cup of pumpkin puree

1 teaspoon of freshly grated ginger

1 cup of unsweetened almond milk

1 scoop of plant-based protein powder

1 tablespoon of honey

**Instructions:**

- All the components should be put in a blender.
- Purée until fluid.
- Enjoy!

Prep Time: 5 minutes

# CONCLUSION

One of the hardest diagnoses a person can receive is a cancer diagnosis. Though receiving this diagnosis can be frightening and overwhelming, it's important to keep in mind that it can be treated and that many people go on to lead active, healthy lives after receiving it. More options than ever are available to assist you in managing your cancer and enhancing your quality of life thanks to advancements in technology and treatments.

The food you eat can be one of the best ways to manage cancer. You can maintain good health and fend off cancer cells by eating the right foods. Newly diagnosed patients can start their journey with recipes that fight cancer. The meals you prepare using these recipes will be wholesome, nutrient-dense meals that will give you the strength and support you need to battle cancer.

These recipes not only assist you in managing your cancer but also give you a way to savor delectable meals and spend time with the people you cherish. You can give yourself the gift of sustenance and joy by taking the time to plan and prepare meals.

Despite the difficulty of receiving a cancer diagnosis, you can fight the disease and lead a full and healthy life with the right diet and support. Newly diagnosed patients can start their journey with cancer-fighting recipes. In addition to giving you the strength and support you need to fight your cancer, they give you a way to take pleasure in scrumptious, nutrient-rich meals and spend time with the people you love.

So don't be afraid to look into cancer-fighting recipes for those who have just been diagnosed if you or someone you know has recently been diagnosed with cancer. You can enjoy delicious meals while fighting your cancer and leading a full and healthy life with the right diet, support, and a little bit of creativity.

Stay steadfast and good luck!